YOUNGER LOOKING SKIN

Younger, Healthier Skin in 4 Weeks

KATE ANDERSON

Third Edition

© 2015

Third Edition

Copyright © 2015 by Kate Anderson
Publishing

Beauty is a kind of radiance. People who possess true beauty, their eyes are a little brighter, their skin a little fresher. They vibrate at a different frequency. We can all look like this. It takes less than you think.

Cameron Diaz

Table Of Contents

INTRODUCTION

Beautiful Skin For Everyone

Growing older can be a great source of anxiety in our lives. Our complexion changes as we age: wrinkles surface around our eyes, mouth and forehead, skin may become dry, oily, puffy, red, or discoloured, we may find hairs where we don't want them. **But all is not lost!**

A few subtle changes to your routine can make a world of difference both to your appearance and your confidence. This does not mean spending vast sums of money or taking hours on beauty routines everyday. It is much simpler than that.

As we age, our skin produces less of the collagen and elastin that give it its tone and suppleness, dead cells are replaced more slowly and blood vessels weaken. But can we really do anything to get younger looking skin? **Yes!**

This simple guide offers top tips on keeping your skin healthy and vibrant from head to toe. In it, you will learn everything from basic care for your skin, hair, teeth, and nails right through to more elaborate beauty treatments and cures common problems like acne, cold sores, and stretch marks.

It is never too early nor too late to start caring properly for your skin. There are plenty of things you can do right now to prevent early signs of ageing and to rescue older, tired looking skin. Unfortunately a lot of bad, in accurate and at times even *dangerous* advice is out there. The aim of this book is to only give you accurate, honest and tested techniques. Now on it's third edition, this book has been updated with the latest discoveries and methods.

Growing older gracefully, with fresh vibrant skin is easier than you might think. This book will teach you everything you need to know.

Let's get started!

Choosing the Right Beauty Products

Don't Waste Your Money!

Standing in the beauty aisle of a pharmacy or department store can be extremely daunting. Not only are there products for every single part of your body, there are also creams, serums, oils, exfoliants, masks, and countless other potions to choose from and they range from the price of a sandwich to the price of a used car!

In my research for this book, I spoke to countless people who told me that almost every month they were trying a new beauty product. Something new they had seen advertised, promising to make them look 20 years younger within 1 day or some other ridiculous claim. And believe me, I am not being all high and mighty here – I myself spent a small fortune on products before I learnt the truth! I hope, with the help of this book, I can stop you from wasting anymore of your money.

But it is not easy to distinguish the rubbish from the effective, I understand. The beauty industry spends *millions* every year on advertising – we are quite literally bombarded day and night with products. Choosing the correct ones is difficult, at first.

Where do you even start?
Which products are worth spending good money on and what problems can be solved for free?
Do these products actually work?

In the next few sections I will discuss a variety of treatments for common ageing concerns and identify when a problem or product is worth financial investment versus those times you really don't need to spend a penny. Lets start with a list of basics must-haves and a few helpful hints to help you find the right products for your skin and your budget.

Basic Equipment

What every woman needs to own

This is your basic list – if you do not own and use the below, this is definitely your starting point. If you do own the below, make sure you actually *use* them! They may be the basics but they are the absolute backbone to keeping your skin fresh and vibrant, even into later life.

Daily Facial Cleanser

You will need a decent daily facial wash as some cheaper products can leave your skin too dry and may cause dry or red patches or a feeling of "tightness"; however, your daily wash should not be a bank breaker.

For skin that's just beginning to show signs of ageing or skin that is in the advanced stages of ageing, I recommend using any daily facial wash containing glycolic Acid. Products with glycolic acid are also great for skin prone to acne breakouts.

A good glycolic wash does not have to be expensive! Shop around to find one that suits your budget and if you're unsure, ask for advice from a sales person or look up reviews online. If you have skin that's sensitive or doesn't react happily to a glycolic acid or other strong chemicals, choose a daily cleanser that uses more natural ingredients or one that is specifically designed for sensitive skin.

Remember to spend your money wisely. Your daily wash is something you will use every single day so by choosing a product in the low to mid level price range you will find that not only is it easy to replace when it runs out, but you will have more cash to spend on more important products.

Day Cream with SPF

Your day cream should be used every morning and should contain sun protection. To choose the right day cream start by reading labels. Look for words like "for oily skin", "for dry skin", "for normal skin". If you're unsure of which bracket your skin falls into, ask yourself questions. Do I sweat a lot? Do I suffer from acne? Does my skin glisten without make-up?

If you answered "yes", a product "for oily skin" will probably by the way to go. If your skin is prone to red patches, dry patches, roughness, or tightness, a product for "dry skin" will probably work best. Also look out for any guidelines on products regarding age.

Many products do specify an optimum age range to help you choose the right level of treatment needed for your age. If you are unsure read the fine print, ask a sales person for help, or check online reviews. Be thorough in your research to avoid spending money on a product that may end up being unsuitable for your skin.

Be sure to test the product on the back of your hand. Choose a product that is light and silky. A day cream that is too thick or heavy may clog your pores and may be uncomfortable for daily use.

Night Cream

Your night cream should again, be purchased based on your skin type. Night creams will be thicker than day creams but shouldn't be too heavy as they may cause break-outs or unwanted morning puffiness.

Remember again to test products on the back of your hand before purchasing to ensure you're choosing the right product and not wasting money on a product that doesn't suit you. If you find the cost of both a day and night cream is too much to spend all at once, use your day cream morning and night until you're ready to purchase a night cream.

Eye Cream

A good eye cream is extremely important! Your eyes are not only the window to your soul, they are also the window to your *age* and your *lifestyle*. You will need a product for morning and one for night or a product that specifies its suitability for both.

Products containing Retinol are highly recommended as they may dramatically repair signs of ageing. However, use care with these products as they can be quite strong and may irritate sensitive or younger skin. If your skin is sensitive or not yet showing signs of ageing, you shouldn't require a Retinol eye cream but using one 1-3 times a week may help to slow down signs of ageing and may also help to boost your confidence.

If your lifestyle involves regular late nights, heavy alcohol consumption or limited and/or odd sleep patterns, having to hand a good overnight revitalising eye cream and/or a morning rescue eye cream will never hurt.

There are many products on the market that will help reduce puffiness and darkness around the eyes which may be more visible after a big night out or a troubled sleep. If you think a product like this is necessary for your lifestyle, I promise you won't regret buying it.

 Top Tip: Apply eye cream with your "ring finger" as is it your weakest finger and will cause less pulling and dragging of the delicate skin around your eyes.

Facial Brush

A motorised round facial brush is a fantastic way to waken up dull, tired skin. Use your brush for a minute or less, 2-3 times per week. Avoid overuse as it may cause skin irritation. Be sure to keep your facial brush clean and dry and replace the brush head regularly.

<u>Your Daily Routine</u>
How to get that vibrant look everyday!

There is no substitute for attentive repetition. Results come from finding the correct path and never deviating from it. Walk that path, everyday.

Edith Bergstrom

It is important to follow a routine to keep your skin in good condition. Not only will it prove to slow down signs of ageing and keep your complexion clear and bright, it may also improve your self esteem and can be a great way to treat yourself after a long day or tough week.

Below, you will find both a simple daily routine to suit everyone and a more elaborate routine for those willing to put in a little extra time when possible. Whatever works for you, try to be consistent and persistent. Do not give up!

There is no over night fix to signs of ageing, but committing yourself to treating your skin nicely will most certainly pay off.

<u>Keeping it Simple</u>

* Wash your face morning and night.

* Each morning apply daytime eye cream, face cream, and a lip moisturiser before applying your make-up.

* Remove your make-up every night – **no excuses!**

* Use a gentle wash before bed.

* Apply nighttime eye cream and face cream.

A More Elaborate Routine

Follow all basic guidelines above and then....

Glycolic peel

For instant rejuvenation of tired, dull-looking skin, use a Glycolic peel roughly twice per week no more than every other month. Glycolic peel kits can have a dramatic effect which is immediately noticeable and long-lasting.

Kits are available in most major pharmacies and beauty supply stores and they can range dramatically in price. Shop around for one that suits your budget and utilise online reviews or advice from trusted friends or family to ensure your money is well spent.

Be sure to read and follow the instructions for your peel kit as they will vary from brand to brand and misuse of these products may cause irritation.

Moisturising Mask Treatment

Use a good quality moisturising mask treatment once a week. The older we get, our skin tends to become more prone to dryness which can leave our faces looking tired and colour-drained. You may find that your skin feels rough or appears saggy.

As we age, our skin becomes thinner and we lose the elastic tightness of our younger days. Poor diet, lack of sleep, medication and illness can also cause dryness and discolouration of the skin. Using a good moisturising mask is a great way to rejuvenate your skin.

Improvements are immediately visible and will therefore leave you feeling satisfied and more confident. If your skin is oily or acne prone, a moisturising mask is probably not necessary and may cause breakouts.

Blemish Focused Face Mask

For younger or oily skin use a blemish focused face mask once a week to help dry out any acne or blemishes. Hormonal changes, medications, poor diet, hot weather, and heavy exercise may lead to oily skin. A good face mask treatment should help to reduce break-outs and can also help you relax and unwind.

For best results use your face mask at the end of the day and remember to use your usual night cream after treatment to avoid drying out.

Rest your eyes!
Rest and cool your eyes throughout the week. Gel masks can be kept in your refrigerator and are a cheap and easy

way to reduce puffiness and dark circles around your eyes.

Gel masks can also be used as a cheap and effective natural treatment for stress, tension and migraine headaches. If you don't want to spend money on another product, use fresh cucumber slices or cold tea bags. Rest for ten to twenty minutes and enjoy some peace an quiet.

Do's and Don't's

Don't make these common mistakes!

The following lists cover steps you can start taking right now to keep your skin looking young and fresh. Start thinking of your body as a machine. **Your face and your body will only perform well and look great if you are giving it the right fuel and the right maintenance!**

<u>DO</u>

* Get plenty of rest.
Do not underestimate the power of "beauty rest". Your skin will benefit greatly from a good sleep pattern. Your eyes will look brighter and dark circles and under eye "bags" will be reduced.

* Drink plenty of water.
What you put into your body will eventually show on your skin. Water will keep you healthy inside and out. It will lessen impurities that are likely to surface as acne and will act as an internal moisturiser for dry skin.

* Eat plenty of fruit and vegetables.
Vitamins and minerals play a big role in maintaining healthy skin, hair, and nails, not to mention keeping your insides happy as well!

* Wash make-up off your face before bed.
Take at least one day a week off from your make-up. Give
your pores a break and let your skin breathe.

* Use sun protection.
We all love the sunshine but unfortunately it does not
love us (at least not our skin!). Use high strength
sunblock to keep your skin safe and healthy. Even if you
"tan well" or aren't prone to sunburn, skin that is
regularly exposed to the sun will age more rapidly than
skin that is protected from it. Wear large sunglasses to
avoid squinting and causing wrinkles around your eyes.
Wear a hat. Invest in a good beach umbrella and use it!

* Wash your face thoroughly after exercising.
Gently cleanse the skin with a wash. Follow up with a
moisturiser which contains ingredients to help to calm
and constrict the delicate capillaries which would have
been busy during your work out. Camomile, acerola
cherry and green tea will all give the skin this support and
come highly recommended.

Be consistent with your skin routines. It may take a
couple of weeks before you see a change in your skin.
Keep at it!

Listen to your skin. If you find a product is irritating your
skin or causing blemishes or breakouts, discontinue use
and find a product more suitable to your skin type and
desired result. Do not continue to use a product that your
skin does not like, change until you get what is perfect for
you.

Thing To Avoid Unless You Want To Damage Your Skin!

This is often the list that people do not want to see. No matter what some magazines and books tell you, there are certain things you just need to ban or at least drastically cut down on, if you want to save your skin. It really is that simple. Sorry to be the barer of bad news! ;)

Smoking

The dangers associated with smoking are well known but cigarette smoke is not only damaging to your health. It also causes unsightly (and avoidable) lines and wrinkles around the mouth and badly stained teeth and therefore can add years to your perceived age. Ask your doctor or pharmacist for help quitting smoking or try to at least cut down where and when possible.

Excess Alcohol

Alcohol dehydrates you, leaving your skin pale and tired looking. It may also lead to poor sleep patterns which will show around your eyes. Keep your drinking controlled for a healthier body and fresher face.

Excess Caffeine

Consuming too much caffeine. Tea and coffee will stain your teeth and dehydrate you. Caffeine consumed late at night may also cause restlessness and poor sleep quality.

Try to keep your caffeine consumption to a minimum and switch to herbal teas in the evening.

Bad Diet

These foods can cause excess oil in your skin which may lead to blemishes.

Excess amounts of salt in your diet. Salt may dehydrate you and lead to puffiness around the eyes and cheeks.

Excess amounts of sugar in your diet. Sugar may lead to tooth decay. Try to keep your intake of refined sugar on the low side.

Processed foods. Frozen convenience foods are full of salt and sugar and may have little to no health benefits. For those of you who are too busy to cook, try to prepare a large amount one or two good quality meals per week, portion out and freeze for days when cooking isn't an option.

Poor Make Up Routine!

Wearing too much make-up or the wrong make-up.
Make-up can clog your pores and cause break-outs and unhappy looking skin.
Choose make-up that is gentle on the skin and be sparing with it. Wearing too much make-up can make you look older rather than younger.

"Overdoing it"

Be careful not to use products that are too abrasive for your skin type or to use abrasive products too frequently. Always read the instructions on new products and follow them.

Rubbing your eyes excessively
Remember the skin around your eyes is very thin and delicate. Be gentle with it!

The Effects Of Too Much Sun

How to enjoy the sunshine without ruining your skin!

This part is so important, both to your health and the look of your skin, that it had to have it's own section! The massive assumption is that you have to live in somewhere like California for the sun to have any sort of negative effect on your skin – **WRONG!** Read on...

Too much exposure to sunlight is harmful and can damage the skin. Some of this damage is short-term (temporary), such as sunburn. However, allowing your skin to burn can lead to future problems, such as skin cancer due to long-term skin damage.

People most at risk are those with fair skin, blue eyes, freckles, and red or ginger hair. People with white (Caucasian) skins have less melanin than those with darker skins, so are at more risk of burning. However, anyone *can* get sunburnt, even those with dark skins and higher levels of melanin.

Short-term overexposure to sun can cause burning. The skin becomes red, hot and painful. After a few days the burnt skin may peel. A cool shower or bath will help. Soothing creams will help. After-sun lotions cool the skin and contain moisturisers (emollients) to counteract skin dryness and tightness.

Sunburn can also result from exposure to other sources of UV light, such as sunbeds or sunlamps!

Repeated exposure to too much sun over a number of years can cause damage to skin. The effects of sun damage include premature skin ageing and wrinkling, brown spots, non-cancerous (benign) warty growths on the skin (actinic keratoses), and skin cancer.

How To Protect Yourself From The Sun

The basic rule is often the most ignored: *avoid the sun when it is strong, cover up, and use high-factor sunscreen!* Some how, this basic advice, is still ignored.

Sunscreens with an SPF of less than 15 do not give much protection. Always use factor 15 or above. Consider a much higher factor if you are on holiday in a very hot country.

Sunscreens can go off and not work after a time. Therefore, do not use out of-date sunscreen (see the use by date on the bottle). Most have a shelf-life of 2-3 years.

Being kept in the sun can cause deterioration of the active protective ingredients in sunscreen. Be wary of buying bottles of sunscreen that have been kept on a shelf in direct sunlight or outside in hot countries. Try to keep your sunscreen somewhere cool and shaded.

Some experts think that the increased use of sunscreen lotions and creams may give a false sense of security. This may encourage people to go into the sun more and, as a result, cause an increase in your risk of developing skin cancers. It has to be emphasised that sunscreen only partially protects your skin.

Using sunscreen does not mean that you can sunbathe for long periods without harm. If you tan then you have done some damage to your skin.

Reflected light can damage too. On sunny days, even if you are in the shade, sun can reflect on to your skin. Sand, water, concrete and snow are good reflectors of sunlight.

Wet clothes let through more UV light than dry clothes. Take spare clothes with you if you expect to get wet.

You can burn in the water. Even if you are swimming in a pool or snorkelling in the sea, you can still get burnt.

Clouds may give a false sense of security. Most of the UV radiation from sunshine still comes through thin cloud. Thick cloud provides some protection, but you still need protection when there is thin cloud.

Many clothes worn in hot weather (such as thin T-shirts) actually allow a lot of sunlight through. You need to wear tightly-woven clothes to protect from the sun's rays. If you can see light through a fabric then damaging UV rays can get through too.

The sun's rays are more powerful at higher altitudes. It may be cooler up a mountain but you will need more skin protection.

Fair-skinned people who sunburn easily are at particularly high risk of developing skin cancer and should be most careful about protecting their skin.

There is no such thing as a healthy tan. A tan is the skin's response to the sun's damaging rays and is therefore an indicator of sun damage.

Artificial tanning from sun-ray lamps and sunbeds is just as damaging as sunshine - so avoid them.

Fake tan from a bottle is safer than a natural tan because no sun exposure is required. Remember that fake tan is not a sunscreen, and, if you plan to go out in the sun, you will need to apply another product. Some fake tans are bronzers that simply stain the skin and can be washed off. Other products contain a chemical that reacts with the skin to give a tanned colour. The long-term effects of these chemicals are not yet known. However, they seem to be safer than tanning in the sun or under a sunbed.

It is not the heat that does the damage but the UV radiation in sunlight, which is present all year.

You can get a lot of exposure to UV doing winter sports, such as skiing, as it is often done in sunny weather and at high altitudes. In particular, remember ice and snow reflect a lot of sunlight. So, you should wear a hat, sunscreen, lip balm containing an SPF, and sunglasses.

Benefits Of Sunshine

Ah, you thought it was all going to be negative didn't you?! ;) Fear not, if you take the proper precautions then sunshine is something you can not only enjoy, but something that can be good for you too!

Sunshine does give one VERY important benefit: Vitamin D!

Vitamin D is vital for good health. Vitamin D is made in the skin with the help of sunlight. Sunlight is actually the main source of vitamin D, as there is very little found in the foods that we eat. This means that to be healthy you need a certain amount of sun exposure.

Sunlight also tends to improve our general well-being and make us happier. It does this by causing us to produce more of a "happy hormone" called serotonin. Physical activities and exercise outdoors are good for us, and we need to balance that against our wish to avoid skin damage and skin cancer. The way to balance the good and bad effects of the sun is to enjoy the sun safely. This means using all the tips above.

So enjoy being out in the sun when it is not so strong. Have short times out in the sun, rather than spending a long time exposed to it, especially in the hotter times of the day and year. When you have to be out in the middle of the day, use protection such as sun creams, hats, clothing and shade. If you want a tanned skin, consider a fake tan cream. Protecting your skin in this way will keep it young-looking and healthy.

Enjoy the sunshine, but keep yourself safe!

Troubleshooting: How To Deal With Things When They Go Wrong

No matter how well we take care of ourselves, there are certain things we simply cannot avoid. Below is a list of solutions to common problems we all face at some point in our lives.

Acne

We all suffer from blemishes from time to time, some of us more than others. Washing your face twice a day can dramatically reduce the severity and frequency of breakouts. Drinking plenty of water and cutting down consumption greasy or sugary foods is essential.

Remove your make up every day or avoid it completely if and when possible so your pores are less likely to get clogged up. Washing your face regularly after sweating at the gym or on a hot day is of upmost importance for acne prevention. If you are suffering from a breakout refrain from touching your face too much as this will add the oil from your hands to the oil already clogging your pores.

Similarly try to keep your hair away from pimples (even though you may want to hide behind it!) as your hair is carrying its own toxins and oils that won't help your breakout. Keep your hair, hands and breakout areas as clean as possible and invest in a cream or gel spot treatment. These products are inexpensive and surprisingly effective. You won't regret buying it.

Top Tip: If you feel like you have a volcano about to erupt out of your face, resist the urge to squeeze it. These types of pimples do NOT respond well to being poked, prodded and squeezed. Leave it alone and it will recede in a day. Mess with it and you'll be stuck with it for at least a week! You can tell what kind of pimple you're dealing with by holding a warm compress to it. If your pimple comes to a head in 10 minutes or so, it's ready for your attention and should respond quickly and easily to light squeezing. If not, leave it alone.**

Cold Sores

No one likes these guys. They can be extremely painful and horrible to look at. If you are one of the chosen few prone to cold sores, taking the herbal supplement Lysine may help in prevention and treatment. Like most vitamins and minerals however, you must be consistent.

Take Lysine daily and you will probably see an improvement to the frequency and severity of your cold sores. When you have a cold sore, start treatment from the moment you feel the tingle. Everyone responds better/worse to different creams and ointments so find what works for you and be consistent. Try the clear medicated patches for when you're out and about.

They are very effective and when covered with lipstick can hide your cold sore so your confidence doesn't take too much of a hit!

Redness Of The Skin

There are many reasons for your skin to become red. Identify the cause of the problem to best take care of it. If you have just begun using a new product, your skin may become red or irritated. Try not to start new products or regimes when you have to work or go out the next day.

If you wake up with an irritated face and you have to leave the house you will likely become flustered and turn even redder so keep new products for the weekends. Leave irritated skin alone! Try not to cover your red face with tons of make up or more products.

It is probably telling you it needs a break. If the redness is causing you discomfort, lay down and relax with a cool washcloth on your face. Keep your alcohol consumption on the lower side as alcohol can cause redness under the eyes and on the nose, some of which may become irreversible over time.

Redness Of The Eyes

Red eyes are usually a sign of tiredness or dehydration so make sure you're getting plenty of rest and drinking plenty of water. Avoid large quantities of caffeine, alcohol and salt. For irritated, itchy, dry eyes, arm yourself with a bottle of "tears naturale".

These are unmedicated eye drops that can be used as often as needed to help moisten your red eyes. They are also fantastic for hiding signs of a late night!

Puffiness

Your skin may become puffy for many reasons. It may be part of a skin irritation from a new or particularly abrasive product or may be caused by poor diet or lack of sleep. Reduce salt intake and increase water intake.

For puffy eyes lay down and relax with cucumber slices placed over your closed eyes for ten to twenty minutes. Alternatively use a refrigerated gel eye mask. Gel masks that cover the whole face are also available and are very useful if your cheeks are also puffy.

Styes

Like cold sores, styes can be very painful and embarrassing and are often the body's way of telling you to slow down. You are more likely to get a stye when you are stressed out or run down. Give your immune system a boost by getting plenty of vitamin C, taking echinacea tablets, and getting plenty of rest.

Avoid touching or rubbing your eyes and ensure that you wash your hands frequently to avoid passing on bacteria and infection to others. Cold, wet tea bags placed over your closed eyes can be very soothing and can actually help treat your stye. Use a medicated cream if necessary. Avoid eye make up and replace any eye make up that may have come in to contact with your stye to prevent reinfection.

Your Teeth, Hair, and Nails: How To Make Sure They Always Look Good

Your Teeth

Taking good care of your teeth will not only prevent painful visits to the dentist, it will also help to keep you looking young and healthy and feeling confident as well as keeping your breath clean and fresh.

You should brush your teeth at least twice a day for two minutes at a time. Using a good quality tooth paste and mouthwash is essential. Flossing your teeth is a must for preventing cavities, gum disease, and bad breath. Try to floss every day or as often as possible. Cigarettes, red wine, tea, and coffee can and will stain your teeth. Try to avoid smoking all together to keep your breath fresh and your teeth clean.

If you love your tea, coffee, and wine too much to give up, brush your teeth after consuming or if that's not possible rinse your mouth out with cold water to minimise staining. Use a whitening toothpaste consistently and your teeth will stay bright.

Top Tip: Smiling makes you look younger! Taking good care of your teeth means you can smile with confidence!

Your Hair

We all have different types of hair and most of us wish we had someone else's! No matter what type of hair you have though, it won't look good if it's greasy, or unkempt. Invest in a decent shampoo and conditioner specifically designed for your type of hair.

Get a new hair do that you love and one that will suit your lifestyle (don't get a hair do that takes an hour a day if you only have fifteen minutes to spare!). Commit yourself to doing your hair every time you're going out. You will feel much more confident if you like the hair on your head and confidence makes you look happy and immediately shaves years off your perceived age.

Make sure to get your hair cut regularly to tackle split ends and product damage. Getting plenty of fresh whole foods into your diet will help maintain the health and growth of your hair.

Your Body and Facial Hair

Body hair can be embarrassing and unsightly and unfortunately as we age, our hormones change and an increase in body and facial hair is to be expected. It is up to you to choose which body hair stays and which goes but here are a few guidelines.

Keep your legs and underarms shaven and your pubic hair tidy at least. Get your eyebrows shaped by a professional and keep up with your treatments. Eyebrow styles can change over the years so avoid doing anything permanent to yours. If you're unsure what you want, ask your beautician to give your brows a natural look. Eyebrows that make a statement aren't usually a safe way to go.

Your upper lip and chin hair will never be in style. Get rid of it! Do not shave this hair though as it will grow back darker and thicker. Laser treatments are a very effective option and the effects last forever but these treatments can be costly, painful, and leave you with a few days of bruising and swelling to deal with.

Waxing is recommended as it can last up to a month and is relatively inexpensive. If your skin is sensitive, inform your beautician and get waxed on a day that you can relax in the house and don't have to face people at work or elsewhere.

Your Nails

The health of your nails may suffer as you age so it is important to look after them. Keep your finger and toe nails clean. If your lifestyle doesn't allow for regular manicures and pedicures, don't worry, you can take care of it at home. Try to avoid biting your nails. This nervous habit can make for very unhealthy looking hands. Use clippers and emery boards to keep your finger nails tidy.

Nails on the shorter side tend to take less maintenance and look better. A coat of clear nail polish can radically wake up tired, neglected-looking hands. Remember to moisturise your hands often. The skin on your hands can betray you as it tends to age rapidly.

Invest in a cheap pair of cotton gloves and wear them to bed after a thorough coat of heavy moisturising cream to keep hands looking and feelings younger.

For your toe nails, follow the same rules. Keep clean and tidy. Avoid wearing ill fitting shoes when possible and see your doctor about any problems you may be having.

Many health issues will cause unavoidable problems with your feet and this can be embarrassing and uncomfortable. These problems can take a lot of time and perseverance to cure so try not to give up.

Your Body: Look Great, With or Without Clothes On! ;)

Your Breasts

You can love them or hate them but you're stuck with the one's you've got so you better make the most of it. The best thing you can do for your breasts is to invest in a few decent bras. Spending a little extra cash is worth it where your breasts are concerned.

The first rule in picking a new bra is to utilise the help of a good bra sales person! Get yourself measured properly every time you buy new bras.

Breast size fluctuates with age, hormonal changes, changes in body weight, etc. Do not assume that you will always wear the same size bra, it's not likely. Try not to be embarrassed when bra shopping and if you are, tell the sales person, they will understand. When trying on bras, use the smallest or middle clasp; not the largest. This not only allows room for your body's subtle changes, but also the eventual stretching of your bra over time.

A new bra should feel sturdy and strong around your back with very little stretching room but it shouldn't pinch or hurt you. The cups of your bra should fit as close as possible against your breasts without being baggy, saggy, or causing your breasts to spill over. Always try your bra on under a top to see how it looks.

For your every day bra remember to choose your bra based on how it looks and feels **under** your clothes (you can always buy different cute and sexy bras for the bedroom!). Remember that bra shopping can be very frustrating. We are all shaped differently so it may take some perseverance finding the right one for your size and shape. Hang in there and trust your sales person.

Other things you can do for your breast health and appearance are a lot less troublesome. Regularly massaging a good quality lotion or oil into your breasts will help with stretch marks and skin elasticity (and might be the kind of thing your partner won't mind helping out with!).

This can help to maintain some lift in your breasts as you age, but even more importantly, touching and massaging your breasts regularly will help you to notice any subtle changes in your breasts that may require the attention of a doctor.

Stretch Marks and Other Scars

Whether yours are the dark red and purple ones or the barely-there white lines, very few of us *love* our stretch marks. Many of us are consumed with negative emotions about them. There are many products on the market that can help reduce the appearance of scars.

I recommend using an oil based product containing Vitamin E, but it's not necessary to spend a fortune on these types of products. Most people will notice the same improvement from regularly applying cocoa butter or even olive oil to their stretch marks. The key is being consistent. Your scars won't disappear if you use a product once.

If you want major improvement you have to commit yourself to using your products daily. If you are the type of person who buys a product and uses it twice, don't spend too much money on a scar treatment product.

The most important thing to remember about your stretch marks and scars is that in most cases, you notice them a lot more than anyone else. The "problem" with stretch marks is that they can drag our confidence through the gutter.

Learn to love your body and your scars and try not to be too nervous or uncomfortable when undressing in front of someone else. Confidence always wins a room faster than fear and awkwardness.

Own your body and be proud of it!

Cellulite

Lumps and bumps have been getting bad press for years but guess what, most of us have them! There are again, plenty of products on the market that target cellulite but in my experience, they aren't necessarily that affective.

Giving the backs of your legs and bum regular massages with oil or lotion can help reduce cellulite (and might be another thing your partner won't mind helping out with!). Alternatively, buy a decent skin brush and salt scrub and give your legs a good vigorous brushing in the shower every day.

Remember: products and regimes are worthless

if you're not eating right and getting daily exercise. Everything you see on the outside reflects what's going on on the inside.

Your Chest and Neck

You may have noticed that as you age, your face elongates and your chin, neck and chest may take on some new features. There are certain signs of ageing that are unavoidable, however, moisturising your chest and neck every day will most certainly slow down the ageing process and reduce the appearance of lines.

It will also help keep the skin of your chin and neck taut by increasing the elasticity in your ageing skin. There are tons of products made especially for this area of the body and many of them are worth the money.

If you don't want to spend a fortune though, stick with a good all over body lotion or cocoa butter and be consistent in your treatments.

Younger Looking Skin: It Is Possible!

This text has covered a variety of tips and steps you can take to prevent and treat signs of ageing. Almost every single part of your face and body has been discussed here and I promise if you take action and be good to your skin, you will see a difference and so will your friends, family, and co-workers.

However, the most important lesson in ageing gracefully is not in a cream or ointment, nor in a pair of tweezers or a waxing strip. The most important thing you can do to look younger and happier is to accept your ageing process as your own.

There is no use reminding yourself or other people about how you "used to" look or what size you "used to" be. You are, right now, the youngest you will ever be. The skin on your face, your chin, your breasts, your hands, your stomach, they are all yours.

There is no need to feel embarrassed or ashamed about the changes affecting your body; it happens to every one of us. So the last tip here, is the most important one I have to offer...

Be Confident

Often times, having a good skin care regime will work wonders on your confidence before changes even take effect. So even if you don't necessarily love every single part of your body, you can feel good about the fact that you're taking good care of yourself.

The easiest and fastest way to look younger is by simply smiling! :)

Printed in Great Britain
by Amazon

36997696R00030